Boost Your Athletic Performance with The Ultimate Guide to Creatine Gummies

By Hugh Webb

Disclaimer:

The information provided in this book is for educational and informational purposes only. The author is not a licensed professional, and the content should not be considered a substitute for professional advice or services. The reader assumes full responsibility for any actions taken based on the information in this book. The author and publisher are not liable for any damages or negative consequences arising from the use or misuse of the information provided. It is recommended that readers conduct their own research and consult with a professional before making any significant changes to their cleaning routine or use of natural cleaning products.

Table of Contents

The Purpose of This Book:

The purpose of this book is to provide a comprehensive guide to creatine gummies as a convenient and effective supplement for athletes and fitness enthusiasts. It aims to introduce the concept of creatine and its benefits, discuss the drawbacks of traditional creatine supplements, and explain the science behind creatine and its various forms. The book also provides information on the benefits and potential side effects of creatine gummies, as well as tips for incorporating them into one's diet and exercise routine. Ultimately, the goal of the book is to inform and empower readers to make informed decisions about whether creatine gummies are a suitable supplement for their personal fitness goals.

Chapter 1: Understanding Creatine

Creatine is a natural compound that is found in our muscles and other tissues. It is made up of three amino acids: arginine, glycine, and methionine. Creatine is an important source of energy for our muscles, especially during short, intense bursts of activity such as weightlifting, sprinting, or jumping.

Supplementing with creatine has become increasingly popular among athletes and fitness enthusiasts as a way to enhance athletic performance and increase muscle mass. The benefits of creatine supplementation are supported by a large body of scientific research.

One of the main benefits of creatine supplementation is increased muscle strength and power. Studies have consistently shown that creatine supplementation can improve performance in activities that require short bursts of high-intensity exercise, such as weightlifting, sprinting, and jumping. This is thought to be because creatine helps to replenish the ATP (adenosine triphosphate) stores in our muscles, which are rapidly depleted during high-intensity exercise.

Creatine supplementation has also been shown to increase muscle mass and improve body composition. This is because creatine can increase the water content of our muscles, which can lead to an increase in muscle size and a decrease in body fat.

In addition to its benefits for muscle performance and composition, creatine has also been shown to have cognitive benefits. Studies have found that creatine supplementation can improve cognitive function, including working memory, processing speed, and mental fatigue.

It's worth noting that creatine supplementation may not be effective for everyone. Some individuals may not respond to creatine supplementation, and others may experience side effects such as gastrointestinal distress, muscle cramping, or dehydration. It's important to consult with a healthcare professional before starting any new supplement regimen, especially if you have any pre-existing medical conditions or take medications.

Overall, creatine is a popular and well-researched supplement that can offer a range of benefits for athletes and fitness enthusiasts. If you're looking to enhance your performance and improve your muscle mass, creatine supplementation may be worth considering.

Chapter 2: Drawbacks of Traditional Creatine Supplements

While creatine supplementation can offer a range of benefits for athletes and fitness enthusiasts, traditional creatine supplements such as powders and pills have several drawbacks that may make them less appealing to some individuals.

1. Inconvenience and taste: Creatine powders and pills can be inconvenient to use and often have an unpleasant taste. Powders must be mixed with water or another liquid, which can be time-consuming and messy. Pills must be swallowed, which can be difficult for some individuals.
2. Digestive issues: Creatine powders and pills can cause digestive issues such as bloating, diarrhea, and gas. This is because creatine can draw water into the intestines, which can cause discomfort and digestive distress.
3. Inconsistent absorption: The absorption of creatine from powders and pills can be inconsistent, which can lead to variability in the effectiveness of the supplement. This is because creatine can be broken down in the stomach and may not be fully absorbed into the bloodstream.
4. Higher doses may be needed: Creatine powders and pills may require higher doses to achieve the desired effects. This is because some of the creatine may be lost during digestion and absorption.
5. Potential for contamination: There is a risk of contamination with creatine powders and pills, as the manufacturing process is not always tightly regulated. This can lead to the presence of harmful substances or impurities in the supplement.

These drawbacks of traditional creatine supplements have led to the development of alternative forms of creatine, such as creatine gummies. Creatine gummies offer a convenient, easy-to-use, and great-tasting alternative to traditional creatine supplements, with fewer digestive issues and better absorption. As a result, creatine gummies have become a popular choice for individuals looking to supplement with creatine.

Chapter 3: The Rise of Creatine Gummies

As discussed in the previous chapter, traditional creatine supplements such as powders and pills have several drawbacks that can make them less appealing to some individuals. This has led to the development of alternative forms of creatine, including creatine gummies.
Creatine gummies are a relatively new addition to the supplement market, but they have quickly gained popularity among athletes and fitness enthusiasts. Creatine gummies offer a convenient and tasty alternative to traditional creatine supplements, with a range of benefits.

1. Convenience: Creatine gummies are easy to use and can be taken anywhere, without the need for mixing or measuring. They can be eaten on the go, making them a great option for individuals with busy lifestyles.
2. Taste: Creatine gummies have a great taste and are available in a range of flavors. This makes them a more palatable option than traditional creatine supplements, which are often unpleasant to taste.
3. Fewer digestive issues: Creatine gummies are less likely to cause digestive issues such as bloating, gas, and diarrhea. This is because they do not need to be broken down in the stomach, and are absorbed more easily into the bloodstream.
4. Better absorption: Creatine gummies are absorbed more efficiently into the bloodstream than traditional creatine supplements. This is because they bypass the digestive system and are absorbed directly into the bloodstream through the mucous membranes in the mouth.
5. Precise dosing: Creatine gummies provide a precise dose of creatine, without the need for measuring or weighing. This makes it easier to achieve the desired dosage, and reduces the risk of over or under-dosing.

6. No risk of contamination: Creatine gummies are manufactured in a controlled environment, which reduces the risk of contamination. This ensures that the supplement is free from harmful substances or impurities.

Overall, creatine gummies offer a convenient and tasty alternative to traditional creatine supplements, with fewer digestive issues, better absorption, and precise dosing. If you're looking to supplement with creatine, creatine gummies may be worth considering as a more enjoyable and effective option.

Chapter 4: Understanding Creatine and its Mechanism of Action

Before discussing creatine gummies, it is important to understand what creatine is and how it works in the body. Creatine is a naturally occurring compound that is produced by the body from the amino acids arginine, glycine, and methionine. It is primarily stored in the muscles and provides energy for high-intensity exercise.

When you exercise, the body uses adenosine triphosphate (ATP) as a source of energy. ATP is quickly depleted during high-intensity exercise, and the body must produce more to continue exercising. This is where creatine comes in.

Creatine helps to regenerate ATP in the body by donating a phosphate molecule to ADP (adenosine diphosphate), which turns it back into ATP. This process provides a rapid source of energy for the muscles, which can improve performance during short, intense bouts of exercise.

In addition to its role in energy production, creatine has been shown to have a range of other benefits for athletes and fitness enthusiasts. These include:

1. Increased muscle mass: Creatine can increase muscle mass and improve strength by increasing the amount of water that is drawn into the muscles.
2. Improved endurance: Creatine can improve endurance by reducing fatigue and allowing individuals to exercise for longer periods of time.
3. Better recovery: Creatine can help to reduce muscle damage and inflammation, which can improve recovery after exercise.
4. Enhanced brain function: Creatine has been shown to improve cognitive function, memory, and overall brain health.

Creatine supplementation has been extensively researched, and numerous studies have shown that it is safe and effective for most individuals. However, it is important to speak with a healthcare professional before starting any new supplement regimen, especially if you have any underlying medical conditions or are taking any medications.

In summary, creatine is a naturally occurring compound that plays an important role in energy production in the body. By supplementing with creatine, athletes and fitness enthusiasts can improve their performance, increase muscle mass, improve endurance, and enhance recovery.

Chapter 5: Types of Creatine and Their Benefits and Drawbacks

There are several different types of creatine available on the market, each with its own set of benefits and drawbacks. In this chapter, we will explore the most common types of creatine and discuss their unique properties.

1. Creatine Monohydrate: This is the most widely used and researched form of creatine. It is the basic form of creatine and is composed of a creatine molecule attached to a water molecule. Creatine monohydrate is effective for increasing muscle mass and strength, improving endurance, and enhancing recovery. However, it can cause digestive issues such as bloating and diarrhea in some individuals.
2. Creatine Hydrochloride (HCl): This form of creatine is composed of a creatine molecule bonded to hydrochloric acid. Creatine HCl is more soluble in water and may be absorbed more easily by the body than creatine monohydrate. It may also cause fewer digestive issues. However, there is limited research on its effectiveness compared to creatine monohydrate.
3. Creatine Ethyl Ester (CEE): CEE is a form of creatine that is made by attaching an ester molecule to the creatine molecule. This is believed to enhance its absorption into the body. However, research has shown that CEE is not more effective than creatine monohydrate, and it may cause digestive issues.
4. Buffered Creatine: This is a form of creatine that is mixed with an alkaline buffer such as sodium bicarbonate. This is believed to reduce the breakdown of creatine in the stomach and enhance its absorption into the body. Buffered creatine may cause fewer digestive issues than creatine monohydrate, but there is limited research on its effectiveness.

5. Micronized Creatine: This is a form of creatine that has been mechanically processed to break it down into smaller particles. This is believed to enhance its absorption into the body. Micronized creatine is effective for increasing muscle mass and strength, improving endurance, and enhancing recovery. However, it may cause digestive issues in some individuals.

In summary, there are several different types of creatine available on the market, each with its own set of benefits and drawbacks. Creatine monohydrate is the most widely used and researched form of creatine, but may cause digestive issues in some individuals. Other forms of creatine, such as creatine HCl, CEE, buffered creatine, and micronized creatine, have unique properties that may be beneficial for some individuals, but there is limited research on their effectiveness compared to creatine monohydrate. It is important to speak with a healthcare professional before starting any new supplement regimen.

Chapter 6: Overview of Scientific Research on Creatine

Creatine is one of the most extensively researched supplements in the sports nutrition field. The majority of studies on creatine have focused on its effects on muscle strength, power, and endurance. In this chapter, we will provide an overview of the scientific research on creatine.

Muscle Strength and Power: Numerous studies have shown that creatine supplementation can increase muscle strength and power. This effect is thought to be due to creatine's ability to increase the amount of phosphocreatine stored in the muscles, which helps to regenerate ATP, the primary source of energy for muscle contractions. A meta-analysis of 22 studies found that creatine supplementation led to an average increase in muscle strength of 8% and an average increase in power of 14%.

Muscle Endurance: Creatine may also improve muscle endurance. One study found that creatine supplementation improved the number of repetitions that could be performed in a bench press exercise by 43%. This effect may be due to creatine's ability to reduce muscle fatigue by decreasing the breakdown of glycogen, the storage form of glucose in the muscles.

Recovery: Creatine may also enhance recovery following exercise. One study found that creatine supplementation decreased muscle damage and inflammation following a high-intensity resistance training session. This effect may be due to creatine's ability to increase the production of certain anti-inflammatory compounds in the body.

Brain Function: In addition to its effects on muscle performance, creatine may also have benefits for brain function. Some studies have suggested that creatine supplementation may improve cognitive function, particularly in tasks that require short-term memory and reasoning skills.

Health Conditions: There is also some evidence to suggest that creatine supplementation may have therapeutic benefits for certain health conditions. For example, some studies have suggested that creatine may be beneficial for individuals with neurological diseases such as Parkinson's disease and Huntington's disease, as well as for individuals with certain muscular dystrophies.

Overall, the scientific research on creatine suggests that it can be a safe and effective supplement for improving muscle strength, power, and endurance. Creatine may also have benefits for brain function and certain health conditions. However, it is important to note that individual responses to creatine may vary, and some individuals may experience side effects such as digestive issues or muscle cramping. It is important to speak with a healthcare professional before starting any new supplement regimen.

Chapter 7: Why Creatine Gummies are a Convenient and Delicious Alternative to Traditional Creatine Supplements

While traditional creatine supplements such as powders and pills have been available for decades, some people may find these products inconvenient or unpalatable. Fortunately, creatine gummies offer a tasty and convenient alternative for those who want to enjoy the benefits of creatine without the drawbacks of other forms. In this chapter, we will explore the reasons why creatine gummies are a convenient and delicious alternative to traditional creatine supplements.

1. Convenience: One of the main advantages of creatine gummies is their convenience. Unlike powders, which need to be mixed with water or other liquids, and pills, which may need to be swallowed with water, creatine gummies can be easily consumed on-the-go without any additional liquid. They can be stored in a gym bag or backpack and easily consumed before or after a workout.
2. Taste: Another advantage of creatine gummies is their taste. Many traditional creatine supplements have a bitter or unpleasant taste, which can make them difficult to consume. Creatine gummies, on the other hand, come in a variety of flavors and are typically much more palatable. This can be particularly important for individuals who have a sensitive palate or are picky eaters.
3. Dosage: Creatine gummies typically come in pre-measured doses, which can be particularly helpful for individuals who are new to using creatine or who are unsure of how much to take. This can help to ensure that individuals are consuming the correct amount of creatine for their body weight and exercise routine, without the risk of over or under-dosing.

4. Absorption: Creatine gummies may also be absorbed more quickly than traditional supplements. Because they are chewable, the creatine is broken down into smaller particles, which may help to facilitate absorption in the digestive tract. This can potentially lead to faster and more effective delivery of creatine to the muscles.

5. Diverse Range of Users: Finally, creatine gummies are a great option for a diverse range of users. They may be particularly helpful for younger athletes or individuals who have difficulty swallowing pills or drinking powders. Additionally, they can be a great option for individuals who are always on-the-go, such as busy professionals or parents.

In conclusion, creatine gummies offer a convenient and delicious alternative to traditional creatine supplements. They are convenient, tasty, pre-measured, easily absorbed and can be used by a diverse range of users. With these benefits in mind, it's clear why creatine gummies are an appealing choice for individuals looking to supplement with creatine.

Chapter 8: Benefits of Creatine Gummies

In the previous chapter, we discussed why creatine gummies are a convenient and delicious alternative to traditional creatine supplements. In this chapter, we will explore the benefits of creatine gummies, including improved athletic performance, increased muscle gain, and improved brain function.

1. Improved Athletic Performance: One of the primary benefits of creatine supplementation is improved athletic performance. Creatine helps to increase the production of ATP, the primary source of energy for muscle cells. This increased energy production can lead to improved performance in high-intensity, short-duration activities such as weight lifting, sprinting, and jumping. Research has shown that creatine supplementation can increase power output, speed, and strength, allowing athletes to train harder and perform at a higher level.
2. Increased Muscle Gain: Another benefit of creatine supplementation is increased muscle gain. Creatine helps to increase water content in muscle cells, which can lead to improved muscle size and definition. In addition, creatine may also help to increase protein synthesis, leading to greater muscle growth over time. This can be particularly helpful for individuals who are looking to build muscle mass, such as bodybuilders or powerlifters.
3. Improved Brain Function: While most people associate creatine with its effects on muscle performance, it may also have benefits for the brain. Research has shown that creatine can help to improve cognitive function, memory, and overall brain health. This may be due to its ability to increase energy production in the brain, as well as its antioxidant properties.

4. Other Potential Benefits: In addition to the benefits listed above, creatine supplementation may also have other potential benefits. For example, it may help to reduce fatigue and improve recovery time, allowing athletes to train harder and more frequently. Additionally, it may have benefits for individuals with neurological conditions such as Parkinson's disease or Huntington's disease, although more research is needed in this area.

In conclusion, creatine gummies offer a range of potential benefits, including improved athletic performance, increased muscle gain, improved brain function, and other potential benefits. While these benefits are not guaranteed for everyone, they are supported by a significant amount of scientific research. If you are an athlete or fitness enthusiast looking to improve your performance, or simply looking to support your overall health and well-being, creatine gummies may be a convenient and tasty way to supplement with this important nutrient.

Chapter 9: Potential Side Effects of Creatine Gummies

While creatine gummies offer a range of potential benefits, they may also have some potential side effects. In this chapter, we will discuss the potential side effects of creatine gummies and how to minimize them.

1. Dehydration: One of the most common side effects of creatine supplementation is dehydration. Creatine helps to increase water content in muscle cells, which can lead to dehydration if you don't drink enough water. To minimize this risk, it is important to drink plenty of water while taking creatine gummies. Aim for at least 8-10 glasses of water per day, and increase your water intake if you are engaging in intense exercise or spending time in hot weather.
2. Digestive Issues: Some people may experience digestive issues such as bloating, gas, or diarrhea when taking creatine gummies. To minimize these side effects, start with a small dose of creatine gummies and gradually increase your intake over time. It may also be helpful to take creatine gummies with food, as this can help to reduce the risk of digestive issues.
3. Kidney Issues: There is some concern that creatine supplementation may be harmful to the kidneys, although research in this area is mixed. To minimize the risk of kidney issues, it is important to stay well-hydrated while taking creatine gummies. If you have a history of kidney issues, it is also important to speak with your healthcare provider before starting creatine supplementation.

4. Other Potential Side Effects: In addition to the side effects listed above, creatine supplementation may also have other potential side effects. For example, some people may experience muscle cramping, although this is relatively rare. Others may experience headaches or nausea. If you experience any unusual symptoms while taking creatine gummies, it is important to speak with your healthcare provider.

In conclusion, while creatine gummies offer a range of potential benefits, they may also have some potential side effects. To minimize these side effects, it is important to stay well-hydrated, start with a small dose, and gradually increase your intake over time. If you have any concerns about the potential side effects of creatine gummies, it is important to speak with your healthcare provider before starting supplementation.

Chapter 10: Choosing a Brand of Creatine Gummies

If you have decided to try creatine gummies as a convenient and delicious alternative to traditional creatine supplements, it is important to choose a brand that meets your needs. In this chapter, we will discuss the factors to consider when choosing a brand of creatine gummies.

1. Quality of the Ingredients: When choosing a brand of creatine gummies, it is important to consider the quality of the ingredients. Look for a brand that uses high-quality, pure creatine and other natural ingredients. Avoid brands that use artificial colors, flavors, and sweeteners.

2. Dosage: The recommended dosage of creatine gummies may vary depending on the brand. Some brands may recommend a higher or lower dosage than others. It is important to choose a brand that offers a dosage that is appropriate for your needs. If you are unsure about the right dosage for you, it is important to consult with a healthcare provider or a fitness professional.

3. Taste: Creatine gummies are designed to be a tasty and convenient way to supplement with creatine. When choosing a brand, it is important to consider the taste. Look for a brand that offers a flavor that you enjoy. Some brands may offer a variety of flavors to choose from, while others may only offer one or two options.

4. Price: The cost of creatine gummies may vary depending on the brand. It is important to consider the price when choosing a brand, but it should not be the only factor. Look for a brand that offers high-quality ingredients, appropriate dosages, and a flavor that you enjoy, even if it may be a bit more expensive.

5. Customer Reviews: Finally, it is important to consider customer reviews when choosing a brand of creatine gummies. Look for brands that have positive reviews from other customers. This can give you an idea of how effective the product is and how it has worked for other people.

In conclusion, when choosing a brand of creatine gummies, it is important to consider the quality of the ingredients, the dosage, the taste, the price, and customer reviews. By considering these factors, you can choose a brand that meets your needs and provides you with the benefits of creatine supplementation in a convenient and delicious way.

Chapter 11: Recommended Brands of Creatine Gummies

If you have decided to try creatine gummies as a convenient and tasty way to supplement with creatine, it can be overwhelming to choose from the many options available on the market. In this chapter, we will provide a list of recommended brands of creatine gummies based on the factors discussed in the previous chapter.

1. Myprotein Creatine Gummies: Myprotein is a well-known brand in the fitness supplement industry and their creatine gummies have received positive reviews for their taste and effectiveness. They use high-quality creatine monohydrate and natural ingredients, with no artificial colors, flavors, or sweeteners.
2. MuscleTech Creatine Gummies: MuscleTech is another reputable brand in the supplement industry and their creatine gummies are a popular choice among fitness enthusiasts. Their gummies are made with creatine HCL and are designed to dissolve quickly in the mouth for fast absorption.
3. Optimum Nutrition Creatine Gummies: Optimum Nutrition is a trusted brand in the supplement industry and their creatine gummies are a good choice for those looking for a high-quality, effective product. They use creatine monohydrate and natural ingredients, with no artificial colors, flavors, or sweeteners.
4. BPI Sports Creatine Gummies: BPI Sports is a well-known brand in the fitness supplement industry and their creatine gummies have received positive reviews for their taste and effectiveness. They use creatine monohydrate and natural ingredients, with no artificial colors, flavors, or sweeteners.

5. GNC AMP Creatine HCL 189 Gummies: GNC is a trusted brand in the supplement industry and their creatine gummies are a popular choice among fitness enthusiasts. Their gummies are made with creatine HCL for fast absorption and are designed to be easy to chew and swallow.

In conclusion, there are many brands of creatine gummies available on the market, but it is important to choose a brand that meets your needs and provides high-quality, effective ingredients. The above list provides a starting point for those looking for recommended brands of creatine gummies based on the factors discussed in the previous chapter. However, it is important to do your own research and consult with a healthcare provider or fitness professional before beginning any new supplement regimen.

Chapter 12: Optimal Dosage and Timing for Taking Creatine Gummies

When it comes to taking creatine gummies, it is important to follow the recommended dosage and timing in order to experience the full benefits and minimize potential side effects. In this chapter, we will discuss the optimal dosage and timing for taking creatine gummies.

Optimal Dosage

The optimal dosage of creatine gummies can vary based on individual factors such as weight, activity level, and overall health. However, the general recommended dosage is 3-5 grams of creatine per day.

It is important to note that some creatine gummies may contain a lower dosage of creatine per serving compared to traditional creatine supplements like powder or pills.

Therefore, it is important to check the label and adjust your dosage accordingly.

It is also important to not exceed the recommended dosage, as this can increase the risk of side effects such as gastrointestinal issues or kidney damage.

Optimal Timing

The optimal timing for taking creatine gummies can also vary based on individual factors and preferences. However, there are a few general guidelines to follow.

Firstly, it is recommended to take creatine gummies after a meal or with a carbohydrate-rich snack. This is because insulin, which is released in response to carbohydrate intake, can enhance the uptake of creatine into the muscles.

Secondly, it is recommended to take creatine gummies consistently, ideally at the same time each day. This helps to maintain a consistent level of creatine in the body and maximize its benefits.

Finally, it is important to stay hydrated when taking creatine gummies, as they can increase water retention in the body. This can help to prevent potential side effects such as dehydration or cramping.

Conclusion:
In conclusion, the optimal dosage and timing for taking creatine gummies can vary based on individual factors, but it is generally recommended to take 3-5 grams per day after a meal or with a carbohydrate-rich snack, at the same time each day, and with adequate hydration. It is important to follow these guidelines and adjust your dosage as needed based on your individual needs and preferences. As always, it is important to consult with a healthcare provider or fitness professional before beginning any new supplement regimen.

Chapter 13: Tips for Incorporating Creatine Gummies into Your Diet

Incorporating creatine gummies into your diet can be a convenient and delicious way to enhance your athletic performance and support your fitness goals. In this chapter, we will provide some tips for incorporating creatine gummies into your diet, including how to use them in pre- and post-workout meals and snacks.

Pre-Workout
Taking creatine gummies before a workout can help to increase energy and improve athletic performance. Here are some tips for incorporating creatine gummies into your pre-workout routine:

1. Take creatine gummies 30-60 minutes before your workout to allow for optimal absorption.
2. Pair creatine gummies with a carbohydrate-rich snack, such as a banana or a piece of toast with honey, to enhance their uptake into the muscles.
3. Consider adding creatine gummies to a pre-workout smoothie or shake for a convenient and tasty boost of energy.
4.

Post-Workout
Taking creatine gummies after a workout can help to support muscle recovery and growth. Here are some tips for incorporating creatine gummies into your post-workout routine:

1. Take creatine gummies immediately after your workout to help replenish your energy stores.
2. Pair creatine gummies with a protein-rich snack, such as a protein shake or a piece of grilled chicken, to support muscle recovery and growth.

3. Consider adding creatine gummies to a post-workout smoothie or yogurt bowl for a convenient and delicious way to refuel.
4.

Snacks

Incorporating creatine gummies into your snacks throughout the day can help to maintain a consistent level of creatine in the body and support your overall fitness goals. Here are some tips for incorporating creatine gummies into your snacks:

1. Keep a pack of creatine gummies in your gym bag or purse for a convenient on-the-go snack.
2. Add creatine gummies to a trail mix or granola bar for a tasty and energizing snack.
3. Consider using creatine gummies as a pre-workout snack to help fuel your workout.

Conclusion:

Incorporating creatine gummies into your diet can be a convenient and delicious way to enhance your athletic performance and support your fitness goals. Whether you choose to use them in pre- or post-workout meals and snacks, it is important to follow the recommended dosage and timing and adjust your regimen based on your individual needs and preferences. With these tips, you can easily incorporate creatine gummies into your daily routine and optimize your fitness performance.

Chapter 14: Sample Meal Plans and Recipes Featuring Creatine Gummies

Incorporating creatine gummies into your diet can be a convenient and tasty way to enhance your athletic performance and support your fitness goals. In this chapter, we will provide sample meal plans and recipes featuring creatine gummies to help you optimize your intake and achieve your fitness goals.

Sample Meal Plans

1. Pre-Workout Meal Plan

- Breakfast: Oatmeal with banana and almond butter, paired with creatine gummies and a glass of water.
- Snack: Greek yogurt with berries and granola, paired with creatine gummies.
- Lunch: Grilled chicken salad with avocado and quinoa, paired with creatine gummies and a glass of water.
- Snack: Hummus with carrot sticks and pita chips, paired with creatine gummies.
- Pre-Workout Snack: Creatine gummies and a piece of fruit.

2. Post-Workout Meal Plan

- Breakfast: Scrambled eggs with spinach and whole grain toast, paired with creatine gummies and a glass of water.
- Snack: Apple slices with almond butter, paired with creatine gummies.
- Lunch: Grilled salmon with roasted vegetables and brown rice, paired with creatine gummies and a glass of water.
- Snack: Protein smoothie with creatine gummies.

- Post-Workout Snack: Creatine gummies and a protein bar.

Recipes

1. Creatine Gummy Smoothie

- 1 cup frozen berries
- 1 banana
- 1 scoop vanilla protein powder
- 1 pack of creatine gummies
- 1 cup unsweetened almond milk
- 1 cup ice

Blend all ingredients together in a blender until smooth. Enjoy as a pre- or post-workout snack.

2. Grilled Chicken and Creatine Gummy Salad

- 4 oz grilled chicken
- 2 cups mixed greens
- 1/2 avocado, sliced
- 1/4 cup cherry tomatoes, halved
- 1/4 cup sliced cucumber
- 1 pack of creatine gummies
- 2 tbsp balsamic vinaigrette

Arrange the mixed greens on a plate and top with grilled chicken, avocado, cherry tomatoes, and cucumber. Add a pack of creatine gummies on top. Drizzle with balsamic vinaigrette and serve.

Conclusion

Incorporating creatine gummies into your diet can be a convenient and delicious way to enhance your athletic performance and support your fitness goals. With these sample meal plans and recipes, you can easily incorporate creatine gummies into your daily routine and optimize your fitness performance. Remember to follow the recommended dosage and timing and adjust your regimen based on your individual needs and preferences.

Chapter 15: Answering Common Questions about Creatine Gummies

Creatine gummies are a convenient and tasty alternative to traditional creatine supplements, but many people have questions about their safety and effectiveness. In this chapter, we'll answer some of the most common questions about creatine gummies.

1. How do creatine gummies compare to other creatine supplements?

Creatine gummies are just as effective as other forms of creatine, such as powders and pills. The main advantage of gummies is their convenience and taste. They are easy to take on the go and can be a more enjoyable way to consume creatine for those who don't like the taste of other forms.

2. How should I store my creatine gummies?

It's best to store your creatine gummies in a cool, dry place, such as a pantry or cupboard. Avoid storing them in direct sunlight or in a warm area, as heat can cause the gummies to melt or stick together.

3. How much creatine should I take and when should I take it?

The optimal dosage of creatine can vary depending on your weight, sex, and activity level. However, a common dosage for adults is 3-5 grams per day. It's best to take creatine gummies around the time of your workout, either before or after, to help enhance your performance and recovery.

4. Are creatine gummies safe for children and pregnant women?

There is not enough research on the safety of creatine gummies for children and pregnant women, so it's best to avoid them if you fall into one of these categories. If you're pregnant or breastfeeding, it's always best to consult with your doctor before taking any supplements.

5. Do creatine gummies have any side effects?
Some people may experience stomach cramps, diarrhea, or nausea when taking creatine supplements, including gummies. To minimize the risk of these side effects, be sure to drink plenty of water and stick to the recommended dosage. If you experience any severe side effects, stop taking creatine gummies and consult with your doctor.

In conclusion, creatine gummies can be a great option for athletes and fitness enthusiasts looking for a convenient and tasty way to consume creatine. By following the recommended dosage and storing them properly, you can enjoy the benefits of this supplement without any major side effects. If you have any additional questions or concerns, be sure to consult with your doctor or a qualified nutritionist.

Chapter 16: Addressing Concerns and Misconceptions about Creatine Gummies

While creatine gummies can be a great addition to your supplement routine, there are still some concerns and misconceptions that people may have about them. In this chapter, we'll address some of these concerns and clear up any misconceptions.

1. Are creatine gummies only for bodybuilders or athletes?

No, creatine gummies can be beneficial for anyone who is looking to improve their performance during exercise. While athletes and bodybuilders may use them more frequently, the benefits of creatine can extend to anyone who wants to improve their strength and endurance.

2. Do creatine gummies cause weight gain?

Creatine itself does not cause weight gain, but it may increase your body's water weight. This is because creatine helps your muscles retain more water, which can make them appear fuller and larger. However, this does not necessarily equate to fat gain. It's important to maintain a healthy diet and exercise routine to avoid any unwanted weight gain.

3. Can I take creatine gummies every day?

Yes, it's safe to take creatine gummies every day as long as you stick to the recommended dosage. Creatine is a naturally occurring substance in the body, so it's not harmful to consume it regularly. However, if you experience any side effects, it's best to consult with your doctor.

4. Are creatine gummies only for adults?

While creatine gummies are marketed towards adults, there are no age restrictions for consuming creatine supplements. However, it's best to consult with your doctor before giving them to children or teenagers.

5.   Do I need to cycle on and off of creatine gummies? There is no need to cycle on and off of creatine gummies. You can take them consistently every day to experience the benefits. However, it's always best to follow the recommended dosage and consult with your doctor if you experience any side effects.

In conclusion, creatine gummies can be a convenient and tasty way to consume this popular supplement. They are safe to take every day, do not necessarily cause weight gain, and are not limited to bodybuilders or athletes. If you have any other concerns or misconceptions about creatine gummies, be sure to consult with your doctor or a qualified nutritionist.

Chapter 17: Summarize the Benefits of Creatine Gummies and Their Potential as a Convenient and Effective Supplement for Athletes and Fitness Enthusiasts

Creatine gummies offer a convenient and delicious alternative to traditional creatine supplements such as powders and pills. These supplements provide many benefits for athletes and fitness enthusiasts, including improved athletic performance, increased muscle gain, and improved brain function.

Creatine is a natural compound that is found in the body and is produced by the liver, kidneys, and pancreas. It is stored in the muscles and helps to provide energy during intense physical activity. Creatine supplements can increase the amount of creatine in the muscles, which can lead to improved athletic performance.

There are several types of creatine supplements, including creatine monohydrate, creatine hydrochloride, and creatine nitrate. Each type has its own benefits and drawbacks, and it is important to choose the right type of supplement for your individual needs.

Scientific research has shown that creatine supplements are safe and effective, and can provide many benefits for athletes and fitness enthusiasts. Creatine gummies are a convenient and effective way to supplement with creatine, and they offer a number of benefits over traditional supplements.

When choosing a brand of creatine gummies, it is important to consider the quality of the ingredients, the dosage, and the taste. Some recommended brands of creatine gummies include Optimum Nutrition, GNC, and Muscletech.

The optimal dosage and timing for taking creatine gummies will depend on your individual needs and goals. It is important to follow the instructions on the packaging and to consult with a healthcare professional if you have any questions or concerns.

Creatine gummies can be incorporated into your diet in a variety of ways, including as a pre- or post-workout snack, or as part of a meal. There are many recipes and meal plans available that feature creatine gummies, and these can provide a convenient and delicious way to supplement with creatine. Some common questions and concerns about creatine gummies include how they compare to other creatine supplements, how to store them, and whether they are safe for children and pregnant women. It is important to do your research and to consult with a healthcare professional if you have any questions or concerns about using creatine gummies. Overall, creatine gummies offer a convenient and effective way to supplement with creatine, and they can provide many benefits for athletes and fitness enthusiasts. By choosing the right brand of supplement, following the recommended dosage and timing, and incorporating them into your diet, you can enjoy the many benefits of creatine gummies and achieve your fitness and athletic goals.

Chapter 18: Encouraging Readers to Try Creatine Gummies and Share Their Experiences with Others

After reading this book, you might be intrigued by the benefits of creatine gummies and wondering if they are the right supplement for you. If you are an athlete or fitness enthusiast looking for an effective way to boost your performance, gain muscle, and improve your overall health, creatine gummies may be the answer.

While traditional creatine supplements such as powders and pills have been around for a long time, they can be inconvenient and difficult to use. On the other hand, creatine gummies are a tasty and convenient alternative that can be taken on-the-go, making them a popular choice among those who are always on the move.

One of the benefits of creatine gummies is that they can help you achieve your fitness goals more quickly and efficiently. Whether you're a professional athlete or a weekend warrior, incorporating creatine gummies into your routine can help you increase your strength, endurance, and overall athletic performance. Additionally, creatine gummies can help you build muscle mass, which is especially important if you are looking to bulk up and increase your muscle definition.

Another advantage of creatine gummies is that they can improve your brain function. Research has shown that creatine can enhance cognitive function, including memory and attention. This is particularly useful for athletes who need to stay focused during training and competition.

If you're worried about the potential side effects of creatine, rest assured that creatine gummies are generally safe and well-tolerated. The key is to follow the recommended dosage and timing, and to choose a high-quality brand that uses pure and safe ingredients.

If you're interested in trying creatine gummies, we encourage you to experiment with different brands and flavors to find the ones that work best for you. Be sure to follow the recommended dosage and timing, and track your progress to see if creatine gummies are helping you achieve your fitness goals.

As you try creatine gummies, we encourage you to share your experiences with others. Whether it's talking to your friends at the gym, posting on social media, or leaving a review on a retailer's website, sharing your experience can help others learn more about creatine gummies and whether they might be right for them.

In conclusion, creatine gummies are a convenient and tasty alternative to traditional creatine supplements. They offer a range of benefits, including improved athletic performance, increased muscle gain, and improved brain function. If you're looking for a way to take your fitness to the next level, we encourage you to try creatine gummies and share your experiences with others.

In conclusion, creatine gummies offer a convenient and delicious way for athletes and fitness enthusiasts to supplement their diet and potentially improve their athletic performance, increase muscle gain, and improve brain function. While traditional creatine supplements such as powders and pills have drawbacks and potential side effects, creatine gummies provide a tasty and easy-to-use alternative. However, it's important to choose a high-quality brand, follow the recommended dosage, and be aware of any potential side effects. By incorporating creatine gummies into a balanced diet and exercise routine, individuals can potentially see a positive impact on their fitness goals. It is recommended that readers consult with their healthcare provider before starting any new supplement regimen, including creatine gummies. Ultimately, with the proper use and precautions, creatine gummies have the potential to enhance an individual's athletic performance and overall fitness journey.

Epilogue:

As you finish reading The Ultimate Guide to Creatine Gummies, we hope you have gained valuable knowledge and insights about creatine and how it can help you achieve your fitness goals.

Our goal with this book was to provide a fun and delicious alternative to traditional creatine supplements, while still delivering all the benefits that this essential nutrient has to offer. We hope that the recipes and information provided in this guide have inspired you to try out creatine gummies for yourself and experience the benefits firsthand.

Remember, incorporating creatine into your fitness routine is just one piece of the puzzle when it comes to achieving your health and wellness goals. It's important to also prioritize proper nutrition, exercise, and rest to optimize your performance and overall well-being.

We would like to thank you for choosing The Ultimate Guide to Creatine Gummies as your go-to resource for all things creatine. We wish you the best of luck on your fitness journey and hope that you continue to prioritize your health and wellness for years to come.

www.ingramcontent.com/pod-product-compliance
Lightning Source LLC
Chambersburg PA
CBHW071028260726
48662CB00024B/2150